THE COMPLETE FIBROMYALGIA GUIDE FOR WOMEN

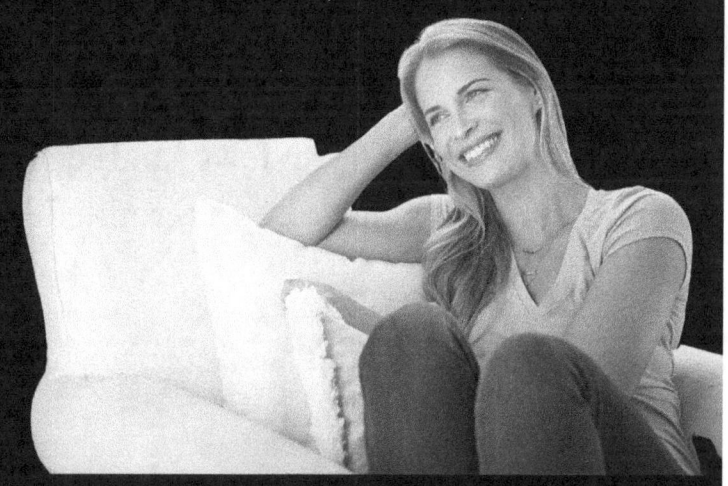

Reverse the Symptoms and Take Back your Life

Dr. Diane Reyes

Table of Contents

Chapter 1: Understanding Fibromyalgia

Fibromyalgia is a complex and often misunderstood condition that affects millions of individuals worldwide, predominantly women. This chapter delves into the intricacies of fibromyalgia, covering its introduction, signs and symptoms, and the diagnostic process.

Introduction to Fibromyalgia

Fibromyalgia is a chronic disorder characterised by widespread musculoskeletal pain, fatigue, and tenderness in localised areas. It is often accompanied by sleep disturbances, cognitive issues, and mood disorders. While the exact cause of fibromyalgia remains elusive, researchers believe it involves a combination of genetic, environmental, and psychological factors.

The hallmark of fibromyalgia is the presence of widespread pain that affects all four quadrants of the body for at least three months. Individuals with fibromyalgia often describe the pain as a constant dull ache, which may vary in intensity. Besides pain, other common symptoms include fatigue, sleep disturbances, and cognitive difficulties, often referred to as "fibro fog."

The impact of fibromyalgia extends beyond physical symptoms, affecting emotional well-being and overall quality of life. It's essential to recognize that fibromyalgia is a real and debilitating condition, despite the absence of visible signs.

Understanding the nature of fibromyalgia is crucial for individuals, healthcare professionals, and the broader community to provide effective support and management strategies.

Signs and Symptoms

Fibromyalgia presents a spectrum of symptoms that can vary in severity from person to person. While pain is the primary symptom, the condition involves a range of associated manifestations:

Widespread Pain: The defining characteristic of fibromyalgia is the widespread pain that affects both sides of the body, above and below the waist. This pain can be migratory, moving from one area to another.

Fatigue: Individuals with fibromyalgia often experience persistent fatigue, even after a full night's sleep. This fatigue can be overwhelming and interfere with daily activities.

Sleep Disturbances: Fibromyalgia disrupts the sleep cycle, leading to non-restorative sleep. Patients may struggle with insomnia, restless leg syndrome, or other sleep disorders.

Cognitive Dysfunction (Fibro Fog): Many people with fibromyalgia report difficulties with concentration, memory, and other cognitive functions. This is commonly referred to as "fibro fog."

Stiffness: Morning stiffness is common in fibromyalgia patients, affecting joints and muscles and gradually improving throughout the day with movement.

Headaches: Chronic headaches, including tension-type and migraines, are prevalent in individuals with fibromyalgia.

Irritable Bowel Syndrome (IBS) and Digestive Issues: Some patients may experience gastrointestinal symptoms, such as abdominal pain, bloating, and altered bowel habits.

Sensory Sensitivities: Increased sensitivity to stimuli like light, noise, and temperature changes is common in fibromyalgia.

Understanding these varied symptoms is crucial for both patients and healthcare providers to establish an accurate diagnosis and develop tailored management plans.

Diagnosing Fibromyalgia

Diagnosing fibromyalgia can be challenging due to the absence of definitive laboratory tests or imaging studies. It often involves a comprehensive evaluation of clinical symptoms and a process of exclusion. The diagnostic criteria, established by the American College of Rheumatology, include:

Widespread Pain: Pain in all four quadrants of the body lasting for at least three months.

Tender Points: Presence of at least 11 out of 18 specified tender points on the body, identified through physical examination.

Additionally, healthcare providers may perform blood tests to rule out other conditions with similar symptoms, such as rheumatoid arthritis or lupus. A thorough medical history, physical examination, and discussions about the patient's symptoms play a crucial role in reaching a fibromyalgia diagnosis.

It is important to note that fibromyalgia is often a diagnosis of exclusion, meaning other potential causes of symptoms must be ruled out. The collaborative effort between patients and healthcare professionals is essential to navigate the diagnostic process and develop a comprehensive understanding of the individual's condition.

In conclusion, understanding fibromyalgia involves recognizing it as a multifaceted condition with widespread implications for physical and mental well-being. From the initial introduction to the intricate signs and symptoms and the diagnostic challenges, gaining insight into fibromyalgia is a crucial step toward effective management and support for individuals living with this chronic condition.

Chapter 2: Demographics and Women's Health

Fibromyalgia is a condition that predominantly affects women, and understanding its demographics and impact on women's health is crucial for a comprehensive approach to management and support. This chapter explores the prevalence of fibromyalgia in women, its impact on quality of life, and the potential role of hormonal influences in this complex condition.

Fibromyalgia in Women

Fibromyalgia has a striking gender bias, with a significantly higher prevalence in women compared to men. According to research studies and epidemiological surveys, approximately 80-90% of individuals diagnosed with fibromyalgia are women. This gender disparity raises important questions about the underlying factors contributing to the development of fibromyalgia, and researchers have been exploring various aspects to unravel this mystery.

Several factors may contribute to the increased prevalence of fibromyalgia in women. Hormonal differences, genetic predispositions, and socio-cultural factors are among the elements currently under investigation. Additionally, women are more likely to report symptoms and seek medical attention, potentially influencing the observed gender distribution of fibromyalgia diagnoses.

Understanding the prevalence of fibromyalgia in women is not only essential for healthcare professionals but also for women themselves. Recognition of this gender-specific pattern can lead to improved awareness, timely diagnosis, and tailored interventions that address the unique needs of women living with fibromyalgia.

Impact on Women's Quality of Life

Fibromyalgia exerts a profound impact on the overall quality of life, and this impact is often more pronounced in women. The chronic nature of the condition, coupled with its diverse and pervasive symptoms, can affect various aspects of a woman's life, including physical, emotional, and social well-being.

Physical Well-being: The widespread pain, fatigue, and other physical symptoms associated with fibromyalgia can limit a woman's ability to engage in daily activities, work, and exercise. Chronic pain can lead to reduced mobility, further contributing to a sedentary lifestyle and potential weight gain.

Emotional Well-being: Living with a chronic condition like fibromyalgia can take a toll on mental health. Women with fibromyalgia may experience heightened levels of stress, anxiety, and depression. The constant management of symptoms and the unpredictability of flare-ups can lead to emotional fatigue and a sense of helplessness.

Social Well-being: Fibromyalgia can impact social interactions and relationships. Women may find it challenging to participate in social events, maintain regular work schedules, or fulfil family responsibilities. The stigma surrounding invisible illnesses can also contribute to feelings of isolation.

Recognizing the multifaceted impact on women's quality of life is essential for healthcare providers and support networks. Tailored interventions, including a combination of medical treatments, psychological support, and lifestyle modifications, can help address these challenges and improve the overall well-being of women with fibromyalgia.

Hormonal Influences

The relationship between hormones and fibromyalgia has been a subject of ongoing research and discussion. While the exact mechanisms are not fully understood, hormonal influences, particularly those related to the endocrine system, may play a role in the development and exacerbation of fibromyalgia symptoms in women.

Estrogen Levels: Oestrogen, a key female hormone, has been implicated in modulating pain perception and sensitivity. Fluctuations in oestrogen levels, such as those that occur during the menstrual cycle, pregnancy, and menopause, may influence the severity of fibromyalgia symptoms. Some women report increased pain and symptom exacerbation during specific phases of their menstrual cycle.

Pregnancy and Postpartum Period: Pregnancy can bring about changes in hormone levels, and some women with fibromyalgia may experience symptom improvement during pregnancy. However, the postpartum period, characterised by hormonal fluctuations, sleep disruptions, and increased stress, can lead to symptom flare-ups.

Menopause: The hormonal changes associated with menopause, including a decline in estrogen levels, can impact fibromyalgia symptoms. Some women may experience worsening of symptoms during this life stage, highlighting the potential interplay between hormonal factors and fibromyalgia.

Understanding the hormonal influences on fibromyalgia is a complex task, and individual experiences can vary widely. Incorporating this knowledge into the overall management of fibromyalgia in women may involve targeted interventions during specific life stages, hormonal therapies, or collaborative care between rheumatologists, gynaecologists, and other healthcare providers.

This chapter provides a comprehensive exploration of fibromyalgia in the context of women's health. From the gender-specific prevalence and its impact on quality of life to the potential role of hormonal influences, this chapter aims to enhance understanding and pave the way for more effective and tailored approaches to managing fibromyalgia in women.

Chapter 3: Causes and Risk Factors

Understanding the causes and risk factors of fibromyalgia is essential for developing targeted interventions and improving the overall management of this complex condition. Chapter 3 explores the multifaceted nature of fibromyalgia, delving into genetic factors, environmental triggers, and lifestyle and behavioural influences that contribute to the onset and exacerbation of fibromyalgia symptoms.

Genetic Factors

Research indicates a significant genetic component in the development of fibromyalgia. Studies have found that individuals with a family history of fibromyalgia are at an increased risk of developing the condition themselves. While there isn't a single gene responsible for fibromyalgia, multiple genetic factors may contribute to its susceptibility.

Polymorphisms in Candidate Genes: Specific genetic variations or polymorphisms in certain genes have been associated with fibromyalgia. Genes involved in the regulation of neurotransmitters, pain perception, and the stress response have been of particular interest. Variations in these genes may influence an individual's vulnerability to fibromyalgia and the severity of symptoms.

Inheritance Patterns: The inheritance of fibromyalgia is likely to be complex, involving a combination of genetic and environmental factors. While having a close relative with fibromyalgia increases the risk, it does not guarantee the development of the condition. This suggests that both genetic predisposition and environmental influences contribute to its manifestation.

Understanding the genetic underpinnings of fibromyalgia provides valuable insights into its pathophysiology. However, the interplay between genetics and other factors remains a dynamic area of research.

Environmental Triggers

Environmental factors play a significant role in triggering or exacerbating fibromyalgia symptoms in susceptible individuals. These triggers can vary widely, and their identification is crucial for developing personalised management strategies.

Physical Trauma: In some cases, physical trauma, such as accidents or injuries, has been linked to the onset of fibromyalgia. The trauma may act as a trigger, activating or worsening symptoms in individuals predisposed to the condition. Understanding the role of trauma in fibromyalgia can help guide preventive measures and rehabilitation strategies.

Infections and Illnesses: Certain infections and illnesses have been associated with the development of fibromyalgia. Viral or bacterial infections can trigger an inflammatory response in the body, potentially contributing to the onset of fibromyalgia symptoms. Exploring the relationship between infections and fibromyalgia may provide insights into preventive measures and targeted treatments.

Psychological Stress: Chronic stress, whether emotional or physical, is recognized as a potential trigger for fibromyalgia symptoms. Stress can contribute to the dysregulation of the body's stress response systems, leading to heightened pain perception and other symptoms. Stress management techniques and interventions may be valuable components of fibromyalgia care.

Identifying and addressing environmental triggers is essential for a comprehensive approach to fibromyalgia management. By minimizing exposure to triggers and developing coping strategies, individuals may experience improved symptom control and overall well-being.

Lifestyle and Behavioral Factors

Lifestyle and behavioural factors, including physical activity, sleep patterns, and coping mechanisms, play a crucial role in the onset and management of fibromyalgia. Understanding how these factors contribute to the condition allows for targeted interventions that can enhance the quality of life for individuals with fibromyalgia.

Physical Inactivity: Sedentary lifestyles and a lack of regular physical activity have been associated with an increased risk of fibromyalgia. Exercise has been shown to have positive effects on pain perception, fatigue, and overall well-being in individuals with fibromyalgia.

Developing tailored exercise programs that accommodate individual capabilities can be a key component of fibromyalgia management.

Sleep Disturbances: Disruptions in sleep patterns are common in individuals with fibromyalgia, and there is a bidirectional relationship between poor sleep and fibromyalgia symptoms. Addressing sleep hygiene, establishing regular sleep routines, and exploring sleep interventions may contribute to symptom relief.

Coping Mechanisms: The way individuals cope with stress and adversity can influence the course of fibromyalgia. Maladaptive coping strategies, such as avoidance or excessive reliance on pain medications, may exacerbate symptoms.

Cognitive-behavioural therapy (CBT) and other therapeutic approaches can help individuals develop healthier coping mechanisms and improve their overall resilience.

Recognizing the impact of lifestyle and behavioural factors on fibromyalgia empowers individuals to actively participate in their own care. Lifestyle modifications, such as incorporating regular exercise and adopting stress-reducing practices, can complement medical treatments and contribute to a holistic approach to fibromyalgia management.

From the interplay of genetic factors to the influence of environmental triggers and the role of lifestyle and behavioural elements, this chapter aims to enhance understanding and guide the development of personalized interventions for individuals living with fibromyalgia.

Chapter 4: Medical Approaches to Fibromyalgia

Fibromyalgia is a complex condition that often requires a multifaceted approach to management. Chapter 4 explores the various medical approaches to fibromyalgia, encompassing medications for symptom management, physical therapy and rehabilitation, and alternative and complementary therapies. A comprehensive understanding of these approaches is essential for individuals and healthcare providers seeking effective strategies to improve the quality of life for those with fibromyalgia.

Medications for Symptom Management

Managing the symptoms of fibromyalgia often involves pharmacological interventions aimed at alleviating pain, improving sleep, and addressing other associated symptoms. While there is no cure for fibromyalgia, medications can help enhance the quality of life for individuals by reducing symptom severity.

Analgesics and Nonsteroidal Anti-Inflammatory Drugs (NSAIDs): These medications are often used to manage pain in fibromyalgia. However, their effectiveness in fibromyalgia is limited, as the condition is not primarily characterised by inflammation.

NSAIDs may provide relief for specific pain-related conditions but are not considered first-line treatments for fibromyalgia.

Antidepressants: Certain antidepressant medications, particularly those belonging to the class of serotonin and norepinephrine reuptake inhibitors (SNRIs), have shown efficacy in managing fibromyalgia symptoms. Duloxetine and milnacipran are examples of SNRIs that may help alleviate pain and improve mood in individuals with fibromyalgia.

Anticonvulsants: Medications commonly used to treat seizures, such as gabapentin and pregabalin, have demonstrated effectiveness in reducing fibromyalgia-related pain.

These drugs modulate nerve signalling and may be prescribed to manage neuropathic pain associated with fibromyalgia.

Muscle Relaxants: In some cases, muscle relaxants may be prescribed to alleviate muscle spasms and improve sleep quality. However, their use is often limited due to potential side effects and lack of conclusive evidence supporting their efficacy.

Sleep Medications: Individuals with fibromyalgia frequently experience sleep disturbances. Medications such as tricyclic antidepressants or certain hypnotic agents may be prescribed to improve sleep quality.

The choice of medications depends on individual symptoms, tolerances, and the presence of coexisting conditions. It is crucial for healthcare providers to work closely with patients to find the most suitable combination of medications to address their specific needs.

Physical Therapy and Rehabilitation

Physical therapy is a cornerstone of fibromyalgia management, focusing on improving physical function, reducing pain, and enhancing overall well-being. Rehabilitation programs are often tailored to individual needs, addressing specific symptoms and functional limitations.

Exercise Programs: Regular, low-impact exercise is considered a fundamental component of fibromyalgia management. Activities such as swimming, walking, and gentle stretching can help improve cardiovascular fitness, reduce pain, and enhance overall function.

Physical therapists work with individuals to develop personalised exercise programs that accommodate their abilities and limitations.

Strength Training: Strengthening exercises, particularly those targeting core and postural muscles, can contribute to better stability and reduced pain in individuals with fibromyalgia. Resistance training is typically introduced gradually to avoid exacerbating symptoms.

Flexibility and Range of Motion Exercises: Improving flexibility and joint mobility can help alleviate stiffness and enhance overall movement. Flexibility exercises may include gentle stretching and activities aimed at maintaining or improving range of motion.

Aquatic Therapy: Water-based exercises, conducted in a warm pool, provide buoyancy and support, reducing the impact on joints and muscles. Aquatic therapy can be particularly beneficial for individuals with fibromyalgia, allowing them to engage in exercises with less strain on the body.

Cognitive-Behavioral Therapy (CBT): While often considered a psychological intervention, CBT can be incorporated into physical therapy for fibromyalgia. CBT helps individuals develop coping strategies, manage stress, and overcome negative thought patterns that may contribute to symptom exacerbation.

Physical therapy and rehabilitation for fibromyalgia require a collaborative effort between individuals, physical therapists, and other healthcare providers. Regular monitoring and adjustments to the rehabilitation plan are essential to accommodate changes in symptoms and functional status.

Alternative and Complementary Therapies

In addition to conventional medical approaches, many individuals with fibromyalgia explore alternative and complementary therapies to address symptoms and improve overall well-being. These therapies, while not always supported by rigorous scientific evidence, may offer benefits for certain individuals.

Acupuncture: Acupuncture involves the insertion of thin needles into specific points on the body. Some individuals with fibromyalgia report pain relief and improved sleep following acupuncture sessions.

The mechanisms underlying its effectiveness are not fully understood, but acupuncture is generally considered safe when performed by trained practitioners.

Massage Therapy: Massage therapy can help reduce muscle tension, improve circulation, and promote relaxation. While the evidence supporting its efficacy in fibromyalgia is mixed, some individuals find massage beneficial for symptom relief.

Yoga and Tai Chi: Mind-body practices such as yoga and tai chi emphasize gentle movements, stretching, and controlled breathing. These activities may contribute to improved flexibility, reduced stress, and enhanced overall well-being in individuals with fibromyalgia.

Herbal Supplements: Some individuals explore herbal supplements such as turmeric, ginger, or omega-3 fatty acids for potential anti-inflammatory and pain-relieving effects. It is important to note that the efficacy and safety of herbal supplements vary, and consultation with healthcare providers is crucial to avoid potential interactions with medications.

Mindfulness and Meditation: Mindfulness-based practices, including meditation and guided imagery, can help individuals manage stress and improve their overall mental well-being. Mindfulness techniques may contribute to better pain coping strategies and reduced symptom severity.

It is essential for individuals considering alternative and complementary therapies to communicate openly with their healthcare providers. While these approaches may offer benefits for some, they should be integrated into an overall treatment plan that includes evidence-based medical interventions.

This Chapter provides a comprehensive overview of medical approaches to fibromyalgia, including medications for symptom management, physical therapy and rehabilitation, and alternative and complementary therapies. The integration of these approaches, tailored to individual needs, is crucial for optimising the management of fibromyalgia and improving the overall quality of life for those affected by this complex condition.

Chapter 5: Lifestyle Modifications

Lifestyle modifications play a pivotal role in the management of fibromyalgia, offering individuals practical strategies to enhance their overall well-being. This chapter explores three key aspects of lifestyle modifications: diet and nutrition, exercise and physical activity, and sleep hygiene and management. Implementing these modifications can significantly contribute to symptom relief, improved functional capacity, and an enhanced quality of life for individuals with fibromyalgia.

Diet and Nutrition

While no specific diet can cure fibromyalgia, adopting a balanced and nutrient-rich eating plan can positively impact symptoms and overall health. Dietary choices can influence energy levels, inflammation, and digestive function, all of which are relevant considerations for individuals managing fibromyalgia.

Anti-Inflammatory Diet: Some individuals with fibromyalgia find relief by following an anti-inflammatory diet. This diet emphasises whole foods, including fruits, vegetables, whole grains, and lean proteins, while minimising processed foods, refined sugars, and saturated fats. Foods rich in omega-3 fatty acids, such as fatty fish and flaxseeds, may have anti-inflammatory properties.

Hydration: Staying adequately hydrated is crucial for overall health and may help alleviate symptoms associated with fibromyalgia. Proper hydration supports joint function, reduces fatigue, and contributes to optimal bodily functions. Individuals should aim to drink an adequate amount of water throughout the day.

Food Sensitivities: Some individuals with fibromyalgia report improvements in symptoms by identifying and managing food sensitivities. Common triggers may include gluten, dairy, and certain additives. Keeping a food diary and working with a healthcare provider or dietitian can help pinpoint potential triggers.

Balanced Meals and Snacking: Eating regular, balanced meals and snacks can help stabilize blood sugar levels and prevent energy crashes. Including a combination of complex carbohydrates, proteins, and healthy fats in each meal supports sustained energy and may contribute to improved mood and cognitive function.

It is essential for individuals with fibromyalgia to consult with healthcare providers or registered dietitians before making significant changes to their diet. Personalised dietary recommendations can take into account individual health status, nutritional needs, and specific symptoms.

Exercise and Physical Activity

Regular exercise and physical activity are integral components of fibromyalgia management, contributing to improved pain tolerance, increased strength, and enhanced overall well-being. While it's important to approach exercise with caution and tailor activities to individual capabilities, incorporating movement into daily life can yield significant benefits.

Low-Impact Aerobic Exercise: Activities such as walking, swimming, and cycling provide cardiovascular benefits without putting excessive strain on joints. Low-impact aerobic exercise has been shown to improve pain, fatigue, and sleep quality in individuals with fibromyalgia.

Strength Training: Progressive strength training, focusing on major muscle groups, can help improve muscle function and reduce pain. Starting with light weights and gradually increasing intensity helps individuals build strength without triggering symptom exacerbation.

Flexibility Exercises: Gentle stretching and flexibility exercises, such as yoga or tai chi, can enhance joint mobility and reduce stiffness. Incorporating these activities into a routine helps maintain or improve range of motion and may contribute to overall symptom relief.

Pacing and Rest Breaks: Pacing is a key concept in fibromyalgia management, emphasising the importance of balancing activity and rest. Breaking activities into manageable segments and incorporating rest breaks can help prevent symptom flare-ups and fatigue.

Individualised Approach: Exercise programs should be individualised, considering the unique needs and limitations of each person with fibromyalgia. Consulting with healthcare providers, physical therapists, or exercise professionals can help develop personalized exercise plans.

While initiating an exercise routine may be challenging for individuals with fibromyalgia, starting slowly and gradually increasing intensity over time can lead to sustainable improvements.

It's crucial to listen to the body, prioritise consistency over intensity, and modify activities as needed to accommodate symptoms.

Sleep Hygiene and Management

Sleep disturbances are common in individuals with fibromyalgia, and addressing sleep hygiene and management is crucial for symptom relief and overall well-being. Creating a sleep-friendly environment and adopting healthy sleep habits can significantly improve the quality of sleep for individuals with fibromyalgia.

Consistent Sleep Schedule: Maintaining a consistent sleep schedule, including consistent bedtime and wake-up times, helps regulate the body's internal clock. This consistency contributes to better sleep quality and improved overall sleep hygiene.

Creating a Relaxing Bedtime Routine: Establishing a relaxing pre-sleep routine signals to the body that it is time to wind down. Activities such as reading, gentle stretching, or listening to calming music can promote relaxation and enhance the transition to sleep.

Optimising Sleep Environment: Creating a comfortable and conducive sleep environment is essential. This includes a comfortable mattress and pillows, minimising noise and light, and maintaining a cool and dark room. Investing in a supportive mattress and pillows can have a positive impact on sleep quality.

Limiting Stimulants: Avoiding stimulants, such as caffeine and nicotine, in the hours leading up to bedtime can prevent disruptions to sleep.

These substances can interfere with the body's ability to relax and may contribute to difficulty falling asleep.

Addressing Sleep Disorders: Individuals with fibromyalgia may experience coexisting sleep disorders, such as sleep apnea or restless legs syndrome. Identifying and addressing these disorders is essential for comprehensive sleep management.

Cognitive-Behavioral Therapy for Insomnia (CBT-I): CBT-I is a structured therapeutic approach that addresses maladaptive sleep patterns and promotes healthy sleep habits. It can be particularly beneficial for individuals with fibromyalgia experiencing chronic insomnia.

Incorporating these sleep hygiene practices into a daily routine can significantly improve sleep quality and contribute to symptom management in fibromyalgia. Individuals should work with healthcare providers to address any underlying sleep disorders and explore additional strategies for optimizing sleep.

We underscore the importance of lifestyle modifications in the management of fibromyalgia. From dietary considerations to the incorporation of exercise and physical activity, and the establishment of healthy sleep hygiene practices, these lifestyle modifications offer individuals practical tools to enhance their overall well-being and navigate the challenges of living with fibromyalgia.

Chapter 6: Mental Health and Fibromyalgia

Fibromyalgia is a condition that not only affects the body with widespread pain and physical symptoms but also takes a toll on mental well-being. This chapter delves into the intricate relationship between mental health and fibromyalgia, addressing the impact on mental well-being, coping strategies, and the importance of seeking professional support.

Impact on Mental Well-being

Living with fibromyalgia can have profound implications for mental health. The chronic nature of the condition, coupled with its unpredictable symptom flare-ups, can lead to a range of emotional and psychological challenges.

Stress and Anxiety: The persistent pain and physical limitations associated with fibromyalgia can contribute to heightened stress levels. Individuals may experience anxiety related to the unpredictability of symptoms and concerns about their ability to manage daily activities.

Depression: The chronic pain and fatigue characteristic of fibromyalgia can contribute to the development or exacerbation of depressive symptoms. The impact on daily functioning, coupled with the challenges of managing a chronic condition, can lead to feelings of helplessness and despair.

Social Isolation: Fibromyalgia symptoms can sometimes limit an individual's ability to engage in social activities, leading to social isolation. The sense of being misunderstood or unsupported may further contribute to feelings of loneliness and withdrawal.

Cognitive Dysfunction (Fibro Fog): The cognitive difficulties commonly referred to as "fibro fog" can impact mental clarity, concentration, and memory. These cognitive challenges may contribute to frustration and a sense of cognitive impairment.

Recognizing the impact of fibromyalgia on mental well-being is crucial for both individuals with the condition and healthcare providers. Addressing mental health alongside physical symptoms is integral to achieving a holistic and effective management approach.

Coping Strategies

Coping with fibromyalgia requires a multifaceted approach that encompasses both physical and mental well-being. Developing effective coping strategies empowers individuals to navigate the challenges associated with fibromyalgia and enhance their overall quality of life.

Education and Self-Awareness: Understanding the nature of fibromyalgia and its impact on both the body and mind is a crucial first step. Education and self-awareness empower individuals to actively participate in their care, make informed decisions, and set realistic expectations.

Stress Management Techniques: Adopting stress management techniques is vital for individuals with fibromyalgia. Techniques such as deep breathing exercises, meditation, and progressive muscle relaxation can help mitigate the impact of stress on both physical and mental well-being.

Pacing and Prioritization: Pacing involves balancing activity and rest to prevent symptom exacerbation. Learning to pace activities and prioritise tasks based on energy levels can contribute to better symptom management and reduced stress.

Cognitive-Behavioral Therapy (CBT): CBT is a therapeutic approach that focuses on identifying and modifying maladaptive thought patterns and behaviours.

In the context of fibromyalgia, CBT can help individuals develop coping skills, challenge negative beliefs, and improve overall resilience.

Social Support: Building and maintaining a strong support network is crucial for mental well-being. Connecting with friends, family, or support groups allows individuals to share experiences, receive understanding, and foster a sense of belonging.

Mindfulness Practices: Mindfulness-based practices, including mindfulness meditation and mindful movement activities like yoga, can promote mental well-being. These practices encourage individuals to stay present, manage stress, and cultivate a positive mindset.

Creative Outlets: Engaging in creative pursuits, such as art, music, or writing, provides an outlet for self-expression and emotional release. Creative activities can be therapeutic and contribute to a sense of accomplishment.

Individuals with fibromyalgia may need to explore various coping strategies to find what works best for them. It's important to approach coping as an ongoing process of discovery and adaptation, recognizing that strategies may evolve over time.

Seeking Professional Support

The complexity of fibromyalgia and its impact on mental health often necessitate professional support. Seeking assistance from healthcare providers and mental health professionals is a proactive step toward managing the emotional aspects of the condition.

Psychological Counseling: Individual or group counseling sessions with a psychologist or therapist can provide a safe space to explore and address the emotional impact of fibromyalgia. Counselling may involve cognitive-behavioural approaches, mindfulness techniques, or other therapeutic modalities.

Psychiatric Intervention: In cases where symptoms of anxiety or depression are significant, psychiatric intervention may be recommended. Psychiatric medications, such as antidepressants or anti-anxiety medications, may be prescribed under the guidance of a psychiatrist.

Pain Management Clinics: Multidisciplinary pain management clinics often bring together a team of healthcare professionals, including pain specialists, physical therapists, and psychologists. These clinics offer comprehensive approaches to managing both physical and mental aspects of chronic pain conditions, including fibromyalgia.

Support Groups: Participating in fibromyalgia support groups provides an opportunity to connect with others facing similar challenges. Support groups offer a platform for sharing experiences, gaining insights, and receiving emotional support from individuals who understand the unique aspects of living with fibromyalgia.

Occupational Therapy: Occupational therapists can assist individuals with fibromyalgia in developing strategies to manage daily activities and improve overall functioning. This may include adaptive techniques, energy conservation strategies, and recommendations for modifications in the home environment.

The decision to seek professional support is a personal one, and individuals should feel empowered to discuss their mental health needs with their healthcare providers. Integrating mental health support into the overall management plan contributes to a holistic and individualised approach to fibromyalgia care.

Chapter 6 emphasises the critical intersection between mental health and fibromyalgia. Acknowledging the impact on mental well-being, adopting effective coping strategies, and seeking professional support are integral components of a comprehensive approach to managing fibromyalgia. By addressing both the physical and emotional aspects of the condition, individuals can enhance their resilience, improve their quality of life, and navigate the challenges of fibromyalgia more effectively.

Chapter 7: Women's Specific Challenges

Fibromyalgia is a condition that predominantly affects women, and understanding the specific challenges faced by women living with fibromyalgia is essential for providing targeted and comprehensive care. This chapter explores women's unique experiences with fibromyalgia, including the impact of the menstrual cycle, pregnancy, and the transition through menopause and beyond.

Menstrual Cycle and Fibromyalgia

The menstrual cycle, with its hormonal fluctuations and associated symptoms, can influence the experience of fibromyalgia symptoms in women. Understanding the interplay between the menstrual cycle and fibromyalgia is crucial for tailored management strategies.

Hormonal Fluctuations: The menstrual cycle involves regular fluctuations in hormone levels, particularly estrogen and progesterone. Some women with fibromyalgia report changes in symptom severity during different phases of the menstrual cycle. Increased pain sensitivity and symptom exacerbation may occur in the premenstrual phase, potentially linked to hormonal changes.

Pain Perception: Estrogen, a key hormone in the menstrual cycle, has been implicated in modulating pain perception. Fluctuations in estrogen levels may influence pain thresholds, contributing to variations in fibromyalgia symptoms throughout the menstrual cycle.

Menstrual Symptoms: The overlap between fibromyalgia symptoms and common menstrual symptoms, such as fatigue and muscle aches, can intensify the overall symptom burden for women. Managing both fibromyalgia and menstrual symptoms may require a tailored approach, considering individual sensitivities and preferences.

Individual Variability: It's important to note that the relationship between the menstrual cycle and fibromyalgia is highly individualized. While some women may experience noticeable fluctuations in symptoms, others may not observe a clear pattern. Tracking symptoms over several menstrual cycles can help individuals and healthcare providers identify potential patterns and implement targeted strategies.

Managing fibromyalgia in the context of the menstrual cycle may involve adjusting treatment plans during specific phases or incorporating additional support during times of increased symptom severity. Open communication between individuals and healthcare providers is essential for optimizing care.

Pregnancy and Fibromyalgia

Pregnancy introduces a unique set of considerations for women with fibromyalgia. While some women experience improvements in symptoms during pregnancy, others may face challenges related to changing hormone levels, physical demands, and potential flare-ups.

Potential Improvement in Symptoms: Some women with fibromyalgia report a reduction in symptoms during pregnancy. The increase in certain hormones, such as progesterone, and changes in the immune system may contribute to this improvement. However, individual experiences vary widely.

Physical Demands: The physical demands of pregnancy, combined with the additional strain on joints and muscles, can pose challenges for women with fibromyalgia. Maintaining a balance between rest and gentle physical activity is crucial to manage symptoms and support overall well-being.

Medication Considerations: The use of medications during pregnancy requires careful consideration. Women with fibromyalgia who are planning pregnancy or are already pregnant should consult with their healthcare providers to assess the safety of medications and explore alternative strategies for symptom management.

Postpartum Challenges: The postpartum period, characterised by hormonal fluctuations, sleep disruptions, and increased stress, can present challenges for women with fibromyalgia. Balancing the demands of caring for a newborn with managing fibromyalgia symptoms requires careful planning and support.

Pregnancy with fibromyalgia necessitates a collaborative approach between women, their obstetricians, and rheumatologists to ensure a comprehensive and safe management plan. Regular monitoring and adjustments to treatment strategies may be required to address evolving needs during pregnancy and the postpartum period.

Menopause and Beyond

The transition through menopause marks another significant phase in a woman's life, and women with fibromyalgia may encounter unique challenges during this period and beyond.

Hormonal Changes: Menopause is characterized by a decline in estrogen levels, which can impact fibromyalgia symptoms. Some women may experience an exacerbation of symptoms during menopause, including increased pain, sleep disturbances, and changes in mood.

Bone Health Considerations: Women with fibromyalgia, particularly those entering menopause, should be mindful of bone health.

Reduced physical activity due to fibromyalgia symptoms and hormonal changes associated with menopause may contribute to a higher risk of osteoporosis. Adequate calcium intake, weight-bearing exercises, and discussions with healthcare providers about bone health are important considerations.

Cognitive Changes: Fibromyalgia-related cognitive challenges, commonly referred to as "fibro fog," may persist or intensify during menopause. Hormonal fluctuations and sleep disturbances characteristic of menopause can contribute to cognitive difficulties.

Psychological Well-being: The emotional and psychological aspects of menopause, coupled with the challenges of managing fibromyalgia, can impact overall well-being.

Women may experience a range of emotions, including anxiety and depression, during this transitional phase.

Navigating menopause and the postmenopausal years with fibromyalgia requires individualized attention to symptoms and considerations. Hormone replacement therapy, if considered, should be discussed with healthcare providers, taking into account both fibromyalgia management and menopausal symptom relief.

In summary, Chapter 7 sheds light on the specific challenges that women with fibromyalgia may face, considering the influence of the menstrual cycle, the unique considerations during pregnancy, and the impact of menopause and beyond.

Tailoring management strategies to address these life phases is essential for optimizing care and improving the quality of life for women living with fibromyalgia. Open communication between women and their healthcare providers ensures a collaborative and personalized approach to navigating these challenges.

Chapter 8: Managing Relationships and Support

Living with fibromyalgia not only impacts the individual directly but also influences their relationships and support systems. Chapter 8 explores the crucial aspects of managing relationships and seeking support in the context of fibromyalgia. This includes effective communication with family and friends, the role of support groups and networks, and the importance of building a supportive environment.

Communicating with Family and Friends

Effective communication is a cornerstone of managing relationships when dealing with fibromyalgia. Open and honest dialogue can foster understanding, empathy, and collaboration among family members and friends.

Educating Loved Ones: Fibromyalgia is often an invisible condition, and loved ones may not fully grasp the extent of its impact. Providing educational materials, articles, or attending medical appointments together can help convey the challenges and complexities of living with fibromyalgia.

Expressing Needs and Limitations: Individuals with fibromyalgia should feel empowered to express their needs and limitations to family and friends. Clear communication about how symptoms fluctuate, the importance of pacing activities, and specific support requirements creates a shared understanding.

Setting Boundaries: Establishing and communicating boundaries is crucial. This may include communicating when rest is needed, specifying how loved ones can assist, and being clear about what activities or events may be challenging. Setting realistic expectations helps prevent misunderstandings.

Emphasising Emotional Support: Beyond practical assistance, emotional support is invaluable.

Expressing emotions, whether frustration, sadness, or moments of triumph, fosters emotional connection. Loved ones who understand the emotional aspects of fibromyalgia can offer empathy and validation.

Encouraging Open Dialogue: Encouraging an environment of open dialogue allows for ongoing communication and adjustments. Regular check-ins, particularly during periods of symptom exacerbation or change, help ensure that both the individual with fibromyalgia and their loved ones are on the same page.

Effective communication contributes to a supportive and understanding environment within the family and social circles.

By fostering open dialogue, individuals with fibromyalgia can build stronger connections and create a network that aids in their overall well-being.

Support Groups and Networks

Support groups and networks provide a valuable resource for individuals with fibromyalgia, offering a sense of community, shared experiences, and practical advice. Engaging with others who understand the challenges of fibromyalgia can be empowering and contribute to a supportive network.

Online Support Communities: The internet provides access to a multitude of online forums, social media groups, and communities dedicated to fibromyalgia. Participating in these platforms allows individuals to connect with others globally, share experiences, and seek advice.

Local Support Groups: Many communities have local fibromyalgia support groups that meet in person. These groups offer the opportunity for face-to-face interaction, fostering a sense of community and providing a safe space for sharing experiences and coping strategies.

Professional-Led Support Sessions: Some support groups are facilitated by healthcare professionals, psychologists, or counselors with expertise in chronic pain conditions. These sessions may include educational components, coping strategies, and a supportive environment for individuals with fibromyalgia.

Family and Caregiver Support: In addition to groups for individuals with fibromyalgia, support groups for family members and caregivers can be beneficial. These groups provide a space for loved ones to share their experiences, gain insights, and access resources to support their role in the caregiving process.

Advocacy Organizations: Various advocacy organizations focus on fibromyalgia and chronic pain conditions. These organizations often provide resources, organize events, and advocate for awareness and research. Engaging with such organizations can connect individuals with broader networks and initiatives.

Participating in support groups not only provides practical advice but also offers a sense of validation and understanding. Connecting with others who share similar experiences fosters a community of mutual support, reducing feelings of isolation often associated with fibromyalgia.

Building a Supportive Environment

Creating a supportive environment extends beyond relationships with individuals and encompasses the broader context of daily life. Several key elements contribute to building an environment that nurtures well-being for individuals with fibromyalgia.

Ergonomic Considerations: Making adjustments to the physical environment can alleviate some of the challenges posed by fibromyalgia symptoms. This may include ergonomic furniture, supportive pillows, and modifications to the home or workspace to minimise physical strain.

Flexible Work Arrangements: For those in the workforce, advocating for flexible work arrangements can enhance overall job satisfaction and performance. Options such as telecommuting, flexible hours, or modifications to the work environment contribute to a more supportive workplace.

Accessible Healthcare: Accessible healthcare is essential for effective management. This includes regular check-ups with healthcare providers, access to specialists, and clear communication about treatment plans. Having a healthcare team that understands fibromyalgia and collaborates on comprehensive care is integral.

Emphasising Self-Care: Encouraging and prioritising self-care practices contributes to a supportive environment. This may involve creating designated spaces for relaxation, incorporating regular breaks, and establishing routines that prioritise mental and physical well-being.

Community Accessibility: Living in an environment with accessible amenities and services enhances overall quality of life. Proximity to healthcare facilities, recreational spaces, and supportive community resources can positively impact individuals with fibromyalgia.

Educational Initiatives: Promoting awareness and understanding within the broader community contributes to a more supportive environment. Educational initiatives, whether in the workplace, schools, or local communities, help dispel misconceptions and create an atmosphere of empathy and inclusivity.

Building a supportive environment requires collaboration between individuals with fibromyalgia, their loved ones, and the broader community. By implementing adjustments and fostering understanding, the overall quality of life for individuals with fibromyalgia can be significantly enhanced.

Chapter 8 highlights the importance of managing relationships and seeking support in the context of fibromyalgia. Effective communication with family and friends, engagement with support groups, and the creation of a supportive environment collectively contribute to a holistic approach to managing fibromyalgia. By fostering understanding, connection, and proactive adjustments, individuals with fibromyalgia can navigate their journey with greater resilience and well-being.

Chapter 9: Balancing Work and Fibromyalgia

Maintaining a successful and fulfilling career while living with fibromyalgia presents unique challenges that require careful navigation and proactive strategies. Chapter 9 delves into the critical aspects of balancing work and fibromyalgia, exploring workplace accommodations, effective communication with employers, and long-term career planning and adaptations.

Workplace Accommodations

Workplace accommodations play a pivotal role in enabling individuals with fibromyalgia to perform their job duties effectively while managing their health. These accommodations can vary widely based on individual needs and the nature of the job but often focus on optimizing the work environment for improved comfort and productivity.

Ergonomic Adjustments: Requesting ergonomic adjustments to the workstation can help alleviate physical strain and reduce the impact of fibromyalgia symptoms. This may include ergonomic chairs, keyboard and mouse modifications, or sit-stand desks to promote a more comfortable and supportive workspace.

Flexible Work Schedule: Negotiating a flexible work schedule can provide individuals with fibromyalgia the flexibility to manage their energy levels effectively. Options such as flexible start and end times, compressed workweeks, or telecommuting arrangements allow for better pacing and reduced commuting-related stress.

Accommodations for Physical Comfort: Accommodations that enhance physical comfort are crucial. This may involve access to a quiet space for breaks, the availability of supportive chairs or cushions, and considerations for temperature control to manage sensitivities to heat or cold.

Job Task Modifications: Discussing potential modifications to job tasks can help individuals focus on their strengths while minimizing tasks that may exacerbate symptoms. This could involve redistributing workload, allowing for task delegation, or incorporating job rotations to manage physical demands effectively.

Assistive Technology: Leveraging assistive technology can enhance efficiency and reduce the cognitive burden associated with fibromyalgia-related cognitive challenges. Employers may consider providing tools such as voice-to-text software, task management apps, or ergonomic computer peripherals.

Job Sharing or Part-Time Arrangements: In some cases, exploring job-sharing or part-time arrangements can help individuals strike a balance between work and health. This approach allows for continued engagement in the workforce while accommodating the need for rest and recovery.

Proactively engaging with employers to discuss potential accommodations fosters a collaborative and supportive work environment. Clear communication about specific needs and potential solutions is essential for successful implementation.

Communicating with Employers

Effective communication with employers is a cornerstone of managing fibromyalgia in the workplace. Open dialogue helps create a supportive atmosphere, fosters understanding, and allows for the implementation of necessary accommodations.

Educating Employers: Providing employers with information about fibromyalgia, its symptoms, and potential impacts on work is a crucial first step. Sharing educational resources or facilitating discussions about the condition helps build awareness and dispel misconceptions.

Clear and Transparent Communication: Transparent communication about symptoms, limitations, and potential challenges is vital. Clearly articulating specific needs, whether related to scheduling, workload, or physical accommodations, allows employers to better understand how to provide support.

Developing a Health Management Plan: Collaborating with employers to develop a health management plan outlines how individuals will address their health needs while fulfilling work responsibilities. This may include discussions about flexible scheduling, designated rest breaks, and strategies for managing symptom flare-ups.

Establishing a Supportive Work Culture: Cultivating a supportive work culture involves fostering an environment where employees feel comfortable discussing health-related concerns. Encouraging open communication, without fear of judgment, contributes to a workplace where individuals with fibromyalgia can thrive.

Providing Regular Updates: Keeping employers informed about changes in health status, treatment plans, or accommodation needs ensures that the workplace remains responsive to evolving circumstances. Regular check-ins can help address emerging issues and maintain a collaborative relationship.

Engaging in Problem-Solving Discussions: Collaborative problem-solving discussions involve exploring potential solutions to address specific challenges. This may include brainstorming alternative work arrangements, adjusting responsibilities, or identifying resources that support both the individual and the employer.

By fostering open communication and a collaborative relationship with employers, individuals with fibromyalgia can create a work environment that accommodates their needs while contributing to the overall success of the organisation.

Career Planning and Adaptations

Long-term career planning and adaptations are essential for individuals with fibromyalgia to navigate their professional journey successfully. This involves strategic decision-making, ongoing self-assessment, and proactive adjustments to align career goals with health considerations.

Self-Assessment and Reflection: Regular self-assessment is key to understanding how fibromyalgia may impact career goals and aspirations. Individuals should reflect on their strengths, limitations, and priorities to make informed decisions about their professional path.

Skill Development and Adaptation: Identifying and developing skills that align with personal strengths and accommodate fibromyalgia-related challenges is crucial. This may involve exploring new skills, adapting existing ones, and seeking professional development opportunities that enhance overall employability.

Networking and Mentorship: Building a strong professional network provides valuable support and opportunities for mentorship. Connecting with colleagues, industry professionals, and mentors can offer insights, advice, and potential avenues for career growth.

Career Flexibility: Maintaining career flexibility allows individuals to adapt to changing circumstances.

This may involve exploring different roles within the same industry, transitioning to part-time work, or considering alternative career paths that better align with health needs.

Entrepreneurship and Self-Employment: For some individuals with fibromyalgia, entrepreneurship or self-employment may offer greater flexibility and control over work conditions. Starting a small business, freelancing, or consulting can provide opportunities for a more tailored and accommodating work environment.

Continued Education and Training: Staying abreast of industry trends and engaging in continued education ensures ongoing professional relevance.

Continuous learning can open doors to new opportunities and enhance the adaptability of individuals with fibromyalgia in a rapidly evolving job market.

Embracing Career Transitions: Recognizing when a career transition is necessary is an important aspect of long-term career planning. This may involve considering changes in job roles, industries, or work arrangements to better align with health needs and career aspirations.

Navigating a career with fibromyalgia requires a proactive and adaptable approach. By incorporating strategic career planning, individuals can continue to pursue fulfilling professional paths while managing the challenges associated with the condition.

In conclusion, Chapter 9 emphasizes the importance of balancing work and fibromyalgia through workplace accommodations, effective communication with employers, and long-term career planning and adaptations. By actively engaging with employers, fostering open communication, and strategically planning for the future, individuals with fibromyalgia can maintain successful and fulfilling careers that align with their health needs and aspirations.

Chapter 10: Advocacy and Awareness

Advocacy and awareness are essential components in the collective effort to improve the understanding, support, and research surrounding fibromyalgia. Chapter 10 explores the significance of becoming an advocate, strategies for raising fibromyalgia awareness, and the importance of active participation in research initiatives.

Becoming an Advocate

Becoming an advocate for fibromyalgia involves actively championing the needs and rights of individuals affected by the condition. Advocacy can take various forms, ranging from personal advocacy within one's social circles to broader efforts aimed at influencing public policies and healthcare systems.

Personal Advocacy: Personal advocacy involves speaking up for oneself and others in daily interactions, whether at work, in healthcare settings, or within the community. This includes effectively communicating needs, educating others about fibromyalgia, and dispelling myths and misconceptions.

Community Engagement: Engaging with local communities, support groups, and grassroots organizations provides opportunities to advocate for fibromyalgia awareness and support. This may involve organizing events, sharing personal stories, and collaborating with local healthcare providers and community leaders.

Online Advocacy: Utilising online platforms and social media is a powerful way to advocate for fibromyalgia awareness on a broader scale. Sharing informative content, participating in online discussions, and connecting with advocacy groups amplify the collective voice of the fibromyalgia community.

Legislative Advocacy: Participating in legislative advocacy involves working to influence policies and regulations that impact individuals with fibromyalgia. This may include advocating for improved access to healthcare, disability accommodations, and increased funding for fibromyalgia research.

Supporting Advocacy Organisations: Many organisations focus on fibromyalgia advocacy, awareness, and research. Supporting these organisations through volunteering, fundraising, or actively participating in their initiatives contributes to a unified effort to advance the cause.

Becoming an advocate requires a commitment to raising awareness, fostering understanding, and actively engaging with various stakeholders to create positive change for individuals living with fibromyalgia.

Raising Fibromyalgia Awareness

Raising awareness about fibromyalgia is crucial to combatting stigma, promoting understanding, and fostering empathy. Effective awareness campaigns can reach diverse audiences, from the general public to healthcare professionals, and contribute to a more informed and supportive society.

Public Awareness Campaigns: Initiating public awareness campaigns involves leveraging various media channels, including television, radio, and online platforms. These campaigns can highlight the prevalence of fibromyalgia, dispel myths, and encourage empathy and support.

Educational Materials: Developing and disseminating educational materials, such as brochures, pamphlets, and infographics, enhances awareness. These materials can be distributed in healthcare settings, community centres, and public spaces to reach a wide audience.

Community Events and Workshops: Organizing community events, workshops, and seminars provides opportunities for direct engagement with the public. These events can feature expert speakers, personal stories, and interactive sessions to enhance understanding and promote dialogue.

Media Collaborations: Collaborating with media outlets, journalists, and influencers can amplify fibromyalgia awareness. Securing coverage in newspapers, magazines, and online publications helps reach diverse audiences and provides a platform for individuals to share their experiences.

Awareness Months and Campaigns: Participating in national or international awareness months dedicated to fibromyalgia, such as May, which is Fibromyalgia Awareness Month, provides a focused opportunity to raise awareness. Planning and participating in awareness campaigns during designated months can generate increased visibility.

Social Media Initiatives: Social media platforms offer a powerful tool for raising awareness. Creating and sharing content, using relevant hashtags, and participating in online challenges contribute to a global conversation about fibromyalgia and connect individuals with shared experiences.

Raising fibromyalgia awareness requires a multi-faceted approach that combines education, community engagement, and collaboration with various stakeholders. By collectively contributing to awareness efforts, advocates can positively impact public perceptions and create a more supportive environment.

Participating in Research

Active participation in fibromyalgia research is fundamental to advancing scientific understanding, improving diagnostic approaches, and developing more effective treatment strategies. Individuals living with fibromyalgia can play a vital role in research initiatives that contribute to the broader scientific knowledge base.

Clinical Trials and Studies: Participating in clinical trials and research studies allows individuals with fibromyalgia to contribute directly to advancements in treatment and understanding. Clinical trials may explore new medications, therapeutic interventions, and diagnostic approaches.

Patient Registries: Joining patient registries facilitates the collection of valuable data on the experiences and characteristics of individuals with fibromyalgia. Registries provide researchers with a comprehensive view of the condition, informing future studies and treatment approaches.

Biobanking Initiatives: Biobanking involves the collection of biological samples, such as blood or tissue, for research purposes. Contributing to biobanking initiatives enables researchers to explore genetic and biomolecular factors associated with fibromyalgia.

Surveys and Questionnaires: Participating in surveys and questionnaires helps researchers gather insights into the impact of fibromyalgia on various aspects of life.

These insights contribute to the development of patient-reported outcome measures and enhance understanding of the condition's complexities.

Advocating for Research Funding: Advocacy for increased research funding is an indirect yet impactful way to contribute to fibromyalgia research. Engaging with policymakers, participating in advocacy campaigns, and supporting organisations that prioritise research funding collectively strengthen the research landscape.

Collaborating with Researchers: Establishing collaborations between individuals with fibromyalgia and researchers fosters a dynamic partnership.

Collaborative efforts ensure that research aligns with the priorities and needs of the fibromyalgia community, promoting more patient-centered outcomes.

Participating in research not only benefits the individual but also contributes to the collective effort to unravel the complexities of fibromyalgia. By actively engaging in research initiatives, individuals with fibromyalgia become key partners in the quest for improved diagnostics, treatments, and overall care.

Chapter 10 underscores the importance of advocacy and awareness in the realm of fibromyalgia. By becoming advocates, raising awareness through various channels, and actively participating in research initiatives, individuals with fibromyalgia and their supporters contribute to a more informed, supportive, and empowered community. The collective efforts of advocacy and awareness pave the way for advancements in research, improved understanding, and enhanced quality of life for those living with fibromyalgia.

Chapter 11: Research and Innovations

Research and innovations play a pivotal role in advancing our understanding of fibromyalgia and improving the quality of care for individuals living with this complex condition. Chapter 11 explores current research trends, emerging treatments, and the crucial role of patient engagement in shaping and participating in fibromyalgia research.

Current Research Trends

Contemporary research on fibromyalgia encompasses a multidisciplinary approach, delving into various aspects of the condition, including its etiology, symptomatology, and treatment modalities. Current research trends focus on unraveling the complexities of fibromyalgia to provide more accurate diagnoses and effective interventions.

Neurobiological Investigations: Advancements in neuroimaging technologies, such as functional magnetic resonance imaging (fMRI) and positron emission tomography (PET), have enabled researchers to explore the neurobiological underpinnings of fibromyalgia. Studies are investigating alterations in brain structure and function, neurotransmitter imbalances, and central nervous system sensitization to better understand pain processing.

Genetic and Epigenetic Studies: Genetic and epigenetic research seeks to identify potential genetic factors contributing to fibromyalgia susceptibility and severity. Investigating gene expression patterns and epigenetic modifications may offer insights into the interplay between genetic predisposition and environmental influences.

Immunological and Inflammatory Pathways: The role of the immune system and inflammatory pathways in fibromyalgia is a focus of ongoing research. Exploring immune dysregulation, cytokine profiles, and inflammatory markers aims to uncover potential targets for therapeutic interventions and enhance our understanding of the condition's systemic impact.

Microbiome and Gut-Brain Axis: The gut-brain axis and the role of the microbiome are emerging areas of interest in fibromyalgia research. Investigations into the composition and function of the gut microbiota aim to elucidate potential connections between gastrointestinal health, inflammation, and fibromyalgia symptoms.

Psychosocial Influences: Research continues to explore the psychosocial aspects of fibromyalgia, including the impact of stress, trauma, and mental health on symptom severity. Understanding the bidirectional relationship between psychological factors and fibromyalgia symptoms contributes to holistic treatment approaches.

Digital Health and Wearables: The integration of digital health tools, such as mobile applications and wearables, is becoming more prevalent in fibromyalgia research. These technologies enable real-time monitoring of symptoms, physical activity, and sleep patterns, providing researchers with valuable data for comprehensive assessments.

Patient-Reported Outcomes: Recognizing the importance of patient perspectives, research increasingly incorporates patient-reported outcomes (PROs). Assessing aspects such as pain, fatigue, sleep quality, and daily functioning directly from the patient's viewpoint ensures a more patient-centered approach to research and treatment.

Keeping abreast of current research trends allows healthcare providers, individuals with fibromyalgia, and their support networks to stay informed about the evolving landscape of fibromyalgia research and potential breakthroughs on the horizon.

Emerging Treatments

The field of fibromyalgia treatment is evolving, with researchers exploring innovative approaches to alleviate symptoms and improve the overall well-being of individuals with fibromyalgia. Emerging treatments aim to address the multifaceted nature of fibromyalgia, combining pharmacological and non-pharmacological modalities.

Pharmacological Interventions: Ongoing research investigates novel pharmacological interventions for fibromyalgia symptom management. This includes the development of medications that target specific pathways involved in pain processing, neurotransmitter modulation, and anti-inflammatory agents.

Neuromodulation Techniques: Neuromodulation techniques, such as transcranial magnetic stimulation (TMS) and transcutaneous electrical nerve stimulation (TENS), are being explored for their potential in modulating pain perception and providing relief from fibromyalgia symptoms.

Mind-Body Interventions: Mind-body interventions, including mindfulness-based stress reduction (MBSR), cognitive-behavioral therapy (CBT), and biofeedback, continue to be areas of interest in fibromyalgia research. These approaches aim to address the psychological aspects of fibromyalgia and enhance coping strategies.

Exercise and Physical Therapy Innovations: Advances in tailored exercise programs and physical therapy interventions are being studied for their effectiveness in managing fibromyalgia symptoms. Personalized exercise regimens that consider individual capabilities and preferences are emerging as key components of treatment.

Nutritional Interventions: Exploring the role of nutrition in fibromyalgia management is gaining attention. Research investigates dietary patterns, nutritional supplements, and the potential impact of specific nutrients on symptom severity and overall well-being.

Complementary and Integrative Therapies: Complementary and integrative therapies, such as acupuncture, massage, and herbal supplements, are subjects of ongoing research. Understanding the potential benefits and mechanisms of action of these therapies contributes to a more comprehensive treatment approach.

Technology-Assisted Interventions: The integration of technology, including virtual reality and telehealth platforms, is being explored as a means of delivering therapeutic interventions for fibromyalgia. These technologies offer innovative ways to enhance accessibility and engagement in treatment.

Multidisciplinary Care Models: Recognizing the diverse nature of fibromyalgia, multidisciplinary care models are gaining prominence.

These models involve collaboration among healthcare professionals from various disciplines to provide comprehensive and coordinated care.

As emerging treatments progress through clinical trials and research validation, they hold the promise of expanding the toolkit available for healthcare providers and individuals with fibromyalgia to tailor treatment plans based on individual needs and preferences.

Patient Engagement in Research

The active involvement of individuals with fibromyalgia in the research process is fundamental to ensuring that research priorities, methodologies, and outcomes align with the needs and experiences of the fibromyalgia community. Patient engagement enhances the relevance and impact of research initiatives.

Inclusive Research Design: Engaging individuals with fibromyalgia in the early stages of research design ensures that studies are relevant, respectful, and inclusive. Input from the patient community helps shape research questions, methodologies, and outcomes that truly reflect the lived experiences of those with fibromyalgia.

Participation in Research Planning: Individuals with fibromyalgia can actively participate in the planning of research studies. This involvement may include contributing to the development of research protocols, identifying relevant outcomes, and providing insights into the practical aspects of study participation.

Collaboration in Data Collection: Active participation in data collection involves individuals with fibromyalgia contributing their perspectives through surveys, interviews, focus groups, and patient-reported outcome measures. This direct involvement ensures that the data collected capture the nuances of the fibromyalgia experience.

Advisory Roles in Research Teams: Including individuals with fibromyalgia in advisory roles within research teams enhances collaboration between researchers and the patient community. Advisory roles may involve providing feedback on study progress, interpreting findings, and offering insights into the implications of research outcomes.

Dissemination of Research Findings: Actively involving individuals with fibromyalgia in the dissemination of research findings ensures that the outcomes are communicated in an accessible and meaningful manner. Patient advocates can play a crucial role in translating scientific findings into actionable information for the broader community.

Participation in Clinical Trials: Enrolling in clinical trials is a direct form of patient engagement in research. Individuals with fibromyalgia can contribute to the development of new treatments by volunteering for clinical trials, thereby advancing scientific knowledge and potentially benefiting from innovative interventions.

Advocacy for Research Priorities: Advocacy efforts led by individuals with fibromyalgia can influence research priorities. By voicing the needs and priorities of the community, patient advocates contribute to the allocation of resources and attention to areas that matter most to those living with fibromyalgia.

Engaging individuals with fibromyalgia in the research process transforms research initiatives into collaborative endeavors that prioritize the perspectives and needs of the patient community. This patient-centric approach ensures that research outcomes have a meaningful impact on the lives of those affected by fibromyalgia.

This Chapter underscores the dynamic landscape of fibromyalgia research and innovations. Current research trends, emerging treatments, and patient engagement in research collectively contribute to advancing our understanding of fibromyalgia and improving the care and support available to individuals living with this condition. By staying informed, actively participating in research initiatives, and fostering collaboration between researchers and the patient community, the fibromyalgia community plays a vital role in shaping the future of fibromyalgia research and treatment.

Chapter 12: Coping Strategies for Daily Life

Effectively managing the challenges of fibromyalgia requires a multifaceted approach that encompasses various aspects of daily life. Chapter 12 explores essential coping strategies designed to enhance well-being, minimize symptoms, and foster resilience in the face of fibromyalgia. The focus areas include time management, stress reduction techniques, and the development of a personalised wellness routine.

Time Management

Time management is a critical aspect of coping with fibromyalgia, as individuals often contend with fluctuating energy levels, pain, and other symptoms that can impact daily activities. Implementing effective time management strategies helps optimise productivity while respecting the limitations imposed by fibromyalgia.

Prioritisation of Tasks: Prioritising tasks involves identifying and focusing on activities that are most crucial or time-sensitive. Breaking down larger tasks into smaller, manageable steps can make them less overwhelming and more achievable.

Setting Realistic Goals: Establishing realistic and attainable goals is key to preventing burnout and frustration. Setting manageable objectives ensures a sense of accomplishment without overexertion, contributing to a positive mindset and sustained motivation.

Pacing Activities: Pacing involves distributing activities throughout the day and week to avoid overexertion. Recognizing personal limits and incorporating breaks between tasks helps manage energy levels and minimizes the risk of symptom flare-ups.

Time Blocking: Time blocking entails allocating specific time periods for different activities. This method helps create a structured routine and ensures that energy is appropriately distributed among various tasks, preventing the accumulation of fatigue.

Utilising Assistive Tools: Leveraging assistive tools, such as planners, calendars, and reminder apps, enhances organisation and time management. These tools can assist individuals in keeping track of appointments, deadlines, and daily activities.

Flexibility in Planning: Flexibility is crucial when managing fibromyalgia, as symptoms can vary from day to day. Building flexibility into schedules allows for adjustments based on energy levels, pain intensity, and other factors that may influence daily plans.

Delegating Tasks: Delegating tasks to family members, friends, or colleagues can lighten the workload.

Communicating openly about limitations and seeking support in accomplishing certain tasks fosters collaboration and eases the burden.

Effective time management empowers individuals with fibromyalgia to navigate daily responsibilities while maintaining a balance that supports overall well-being.

Stress Reduction Techniques

Stress management is integral to coping with fibromyalgia, as stress can exacerbate symptoms and contribute to a cycle of increased pain and discomfort. Implementing stress reduction techniques promotes emotional well-being and helps break the link between stress and fibromyalgia symptoms.

Mindfulness and Meditation: Mindfulness practices, including meditation and deep-breathing exercises, can alleviate stress and promote relaxation. Mindfulness encourages individuals to focus on the present moment, fostering a sense of calm and reducing the impact of stressors.

Progressive Muscle Relaxation (PMR): PMR involves systematically tensing and then relaxing different muscle groups to release tension. This technique helps individuals become more aware of physical sensations and actively relax the body, reducing overall stress levels.

Yoga and Tai Chi: Gentle forms of exercise, such as yoga and tai chi, combine physical activity with mindfulness. These practices enhance flexibility, improve balance, and contribute to stress reduction through the integration of breath and movement.

Cognitive-Behavioral Therapy (CBT): CBT is a therapeutic approach that addresses the relationship between thoughts, feelings, and behaviours.

Learning cognitive restructuring techniques helps individuals reframe negative thought patterns and manage stress more effectively.

Artistic Expression: Engaging in creative pursuits, such as art, music, or writing, provides a channel for self-expression and stress relief. Artistic activities can be therapeutic, offering a means to express emotions and cope with the challenges of fibromyalgia.

Nature and Outdoor Activities: Spending time in nature and engaging in outdoor activities can have a positive impact on stress levels. Whether it's a leisurely walk in the park, gardening, or simply enjoying natural surroundings, outdoor experiences contribute to overall well-being.

Aromatherapy: Aromatherapy involves the use of scents, such as essential oils, to promote relaxation and alleviate stress. Scents like lavender, chamomile, and eucalyptus are known for their calming properties and can be incorporated into daily routines.

Social Support: Maintaining strong social connections provides a valuable buffer against stress. Sharing experiences, seeking emotional support, and staying connected with friends and family foster a sense of belonging and contribute to emotional resilience.

Stress reduction techniques are essential tools for individuals with fibromyalgia to manage the emotional and physical toll of stressors, ultimately improving overall quality of life.

Creating a Wellness Routine

Establishing a personalised wellness routine is central to managing fibromyalgia and promoting holistic well-being. A comprehensive wellness routine encompasses various self-care practices that address physical, mental, and emotional aspects of health.

Regular Exercise: Incorporating regular, gentle exercise into a wellness routine is crucial for managing fibromyalgia symptoms. Low-impact activities such as walking, swimming, or cycling contribute to overall fitness and can enhance mood and energy levels.

Balanced Nutrition: Adopting a balanced and nutritious diet supports overall health and can influence fibromyalgia symptoms. Including a variety of fruits, vegetables, lean proteins, and whole grains contributes to optimal nutrition and energy levels.

Adequate Sleep Hygiene: Prioritizing good sleep hygiene is essential for individuals with fibromyalgia. Creating a sleep-conducive environment, adhering to a consistent sleep schedule, and incorporating relaxation techniques contribute to improved sleep quality.

Hydration: Staying adequately hydrated is crucial for overall health. Proper hydration supports bodily functions, helps manage fatigue, and may contribute to the reduction of certain symptoms associated with fibromyalgia.

Stress-Reduction Practices: Integrating stress-reduction practices into a wellness routine enhances emotional well-being. This may include mindfulness exercises, relaxation techniques, and activities that promote a sense of calm and balance.

Pacing and Rest: Incorporating pacing strategies and scheduled rest breaks into daily routines prevents overexertion and minimizes the risk of symptom flare-ups. Balancing activity with periods of rest is essential for managing fibromyalgia effectively.

Mind-Body Practices: Mind-body practices, such as meditation, guided imagery, or progressive muscle relaxation, contribute to mental and emotional well-being. These practices foster a connection between the mind and body, promoting relaxation and resilience.

Holistic Therapies: Exploring holistic therapies, such as acupuncture, massage, or chiropractic care, can complement conventional medical approaches. These therapies may provide relief from specific symptoms and contribute to an overall sense of well-being.

Hobbies and Leisure Activities: Engaging in hobbies and leisure activities that bring joy and fulfilment contributes to a balanced and fulfilling life. Whether it's reading, gardening, crafting, or pursuing artistic endeavors, these activities enhance overall well-being.

Creating a personalised wellness routine requires experimentation and adaptation to individual preferences and needs. By integrating these elements into daily life, individuals with fibromyalgia can actively contribute to their overall health and resilience.

In conclusion, this Chapter emphasises coping strategies for daily life that are essential for individuals living with fibromyalgia. Time management, stress reduction techniques, and the development of a personalised wellness routine collectively contribute to the effective management of symptoms, enhancement of well-being, and the cultivation of resilience in the face of fibromyalgia.

By incorporating these strategies into daily routines, individuals can navigate the challenges of fibromyalgia with greater ease and foster a holistic approach to health and wellness.

Chapter 13: Navigating the Healthcare System

Navigating the healthcare system is a crucial aspect of managing fibromyalgia effectively. Chapter 13 addresses key elements in this process, offering guidance on communicating with healthcare providers, understanding insurance and financial considerations, and advocating for patient rights within the healthcare system.

Communicating with Healthcare Providers

Effective communication with healthcare providers is fundamental to receiving quality care and managing fibromyalgia successfully. Open and clear communication fosters a collaborative relationship between individuals with fibromyalgia and their healthcare team.

Preparation for Appointments: Prior to appointments, individuals should prepare a list of symptoms, questions, and any changes in their condition. This ensures that all relevant information is communicated during the limited time of the appointment.

Open and Honest Communication: Openness and honesty about symptoms, concerns, and treatment preferences create a foundation for effective communication. Clearly expressing the impact of fibromyalgia on daily life helps providers tailor treatment plans to individual needs.

Active Participation in Decision-Making: Actively participating in treatment decisions involves discussing options, potential benefits, and risks with healthcare providers. Individuals with fibromyalgia should feel empowered to voice their preferences and concerns, contributing to shared decision-making.

Seeking Clarification: If there are uncertainties or unfamiliar terms during discussions, individuals should seek clarification from their healthcare providers. Understanding the rationale behind treatment recommendations and the expected outcomes is essential for informed decision-making.

Maintaining a Symptom Journal: Keeping a symptom journal helps individuals track changes in symptoms, identify triggers, and provide healthcare providers with a comprehensive overview of their condition. This tool aids in more accurate diagnosis and treatment adjustments.

Utilizing Technology: Leveraging technology, such as secure messaging platforms or patient portals, facilitates ongoing communication between appointments. This allows individuals to share updates, ask questions, and receive guidance from their healthcare team.

Building a Long-Term Relationship: Building a long-term relationship with healthcare providers promotes continuity of care. Regular check-ins, follow-up appointments, and periodic reviews of treatment plans contribute to ongoing support and adjustments as needed.

Advocating for Comprehensive Care: Individuals with fibromyalgia should advocate for comprehensive care that considers the multidimensional aspects of the condition. This may involve collaboration with specialists, therapists, and other healthcare professionals to address physical, mental, and emotional well-being.

Effective communication with healthcare providers establishes a collaborative and supportive environment, ensuring that individuals with fibromyalgia receive personalised and comprehensive care.

Insurance and Financial Considerations

Understanding insurance and financial considerations is essential for individuals with fibromyalgia to access necessary medical care and manage associated costs. Navigating insurance policies, handling financial challenges, and advocating for coverage are crucial components of this process.

Reviewing Insurance Coverage: Individuals should thoroughly review their insurance policies to understand coverage for fibromyalgia-related treatments, medications, and healthcare services. Being aware of limitations, copayments, deductibles, and coverage exclusions helps prevent financial surprises.

Communicating with Insurance Providers: Clear communication with insurance providers is vital. Individuals can inquire about coverage details, obtain pre-authorization for treatments, and seek clarification on billing matters. Advocating for necessary treatments ensures that insurance is utilised to its fullest extent.

Exploring Prescription Assistance Programs: For medications prescribed for fibromyalgia, exploring prescription assistance programs or patient assistance programs provided by pharmaceutical companies can help offset costs. These programs may offer discounts or financial assistance for eligible individuals.

Understanding Flexible Spending Accounts (FSAs) and Health Savings Accounts (HSAs): Individuals with access to FSAs or HSAs should understand how these accounts can be utilized to cover eligible medical expenses. These accounts may allow for tax-free contributions and withdrawals for qualified healthcare expenses.

Financial Planning for Treatment Costs: Anticipating and planning for treatment costs involves creating a budget that considers medical expenses related to fibromyalgia. Prioritising essential treatments, exploring cost-saving measures, and seeking financial advice can contribute to effective financial planning.

Appealing Insurance Denials: If insurance claims are denied, individuals have the right to appeal these decisions. Understanding the appeals process, gathering supporting documentation, and working with healthcare providers can improve the chances of successful appeals.

Exploring Alternative Therapies: Exploring alternative therapies that may not be covered by insurance requires careful consideration of associated costs. Individuals should weigh the potential benefits against the financial implications and discuss options with their healthcare providers.

Seeking Financial Assistance: Financial assistance programs, nonprofit organisations, and community resources may provide support for individuals facing financial challenges related to fibromyalgia. Researching available assistance options and reaching out to relevant organisations can offer valuable assistance.

Navigating insurance and financial considerations requires proactive engagement, advocacy, and careful planning to ensure that individuals with fibromyalgia can access the necessary care and support without undue financial strain.

Patient Rights and Advocacy

Understanding patient rights and actively engaging in advocacy are integral to ensuring individuals with fibromyalgia receive fair and equitable treatment within the healthcare system. Advocacy efforts can contribute to policy changes, increased awareness, and improved access to quality care.

Knowing Patient Rights: Individuals with fibromyalgia should be aware of their rights as patients. This includes the right to informed consent, privacy, and the right to receive respectful and nondiscriminatory care. Understanding these rights empowers individuals to advocate for themselves.

Participating in Shared Decision-Making: Shared decision-making involves collaborative discussions between patients and healthcare providers about treatment options, risks, and benefits. Actively participating in these discussions ensures that individuals have a say in their care and treatment plans.

Advocating for Accessible Healthcare: Advocacy for accessible healthcare involves raising awareness about the unique needs of individuals with fibromyalgia and promoting policies that enhance accessibility. This may include advocating for accommodations, pain management strategies, and disability support.

Fighting Stigma and Discrimination: Advocating against stigma and discrimination involves challenging misconceptions about fibromyalgia and ensuring that individuals with the condition are treated with dignity and respect. This may involve education campaigns, community outreach, and collaboration with advocacy organizations.

Joining Patient Advocacy Groups: Patient advocacy groups focus on raising awareness, promoting research, and advocating for policy changes related to fibromyalgia. Joining these groups provides individuals with a platform to contribute to collective advocacy efforts and stay informed about relevant issues.

Engaging in Legislative Advocacy: Legislative advocacy involves actively participating in efforts to shape healthcare policies that impact individuals with fibromyalgia.

This may include contacting legislators, participating in advocacy campaigns, and supporting initiatives that address the needs of the fibromyalgia community.

Promoting Research Funding: Advocating for increased research funding for fibromyalgia is essential to advancing scientific understanding and improving treatment options. Individuals can engage in advocacy efforts that emphasize the importance of funding for research initiatives.

Educating Healthcare Providers: Educating healthcare providers about fibromyalgia is a form of advocacy that contributes to improved understanding and more informed care.

Sharing reliable information, personal experiences, and resources with healthcare professionals fosters a collaborative approach to treatment.

Patient rights and advocacy are interconnected, empowering individuals with fibromyalgia to actively shape their healthcare experiences and contribute to positive changes within the broader healthcare system.

Chapter 13 provides valuable insights into navigating the healthcare system for individuals with fibromyalgia. Effective communication with healthcare providers, understanding insurance and financial considerations, and advocating for patient rights collectively contribute to a comprehensive approach to managing fibromyalgia within the healthcare landscape. By actively engaging in these aspects, individuals can enhance their overall healthcare experience, access necessary treatments, and contribute to broader efforts to improve fibromyalgia care and support.

Chapter 14: Future Outlook and Hope

Navigating the landscape of fibromyalgia involves not only understanding the present challenges but also looking towards the future with optimism. Chapter 14 explores the promising aspects of fibromyalgia, including advances in research, personal stories of triumph, and strategies for building a positive outlook.

Advances in Fibromyalgia Research

The field of fibromyalgia research is dynamic, with ongoing efforts aimed at unravelling the complexities of the condition and improving treatment options. Advances in research contribute to a more nuanced understanding of fibromyalgia, offering hope for enhanced diagnostics, targeted therapies, and improved overall care.

Biomarker Discovery: Identifying reliable biomarkers for fibromyalgia is a priority in current research. Biomarkers are measurable indicators that can assist in the diagnosis and monitoring of the condition. The discovery of specific biomarkers may lead to more accurate and objective diagnostic criteria.

Precision Medicine Approaches: The concept of precision medicine involves tailoring treatments to individual characteristics, such as genetic makeup, lifestyle factors, and symptom profiles. Advances in precision medicine may lead to more personalized and effective interventions for individuals with fibromyalgia.

Neurobiological Insights: Ongoing neurobiological research aims to uncover the underlying mechanisms of pain perception and central sensitization in fibromyalgia. Understanding these processes at the molecular and cellular levels may pave the way for targeted therapies that address the root causes of fibromyalgia symptoms.

Innovations in Pain Management: Research into innovative pain management strategies is a focal point. This includes the development of medications with fewer side effects, neuromodulation techniques, and novel approaches to modulating pain pathways. Advancements in pain management contribute to improved quality of life for individuals with fibromyalgia.

Psychosocial Interventions: The integration of psychosocial interventions, such as cognitive-behavioral therapy (CBT) and mindfulness-based approaches, continues to be an area of active research. Understanding the impact of psychological factors on fibromyalgia and refining therapeutic interventions enhances comprehensive care.

Patient-Reported Outcomes Research: Emphasising the importance of patient perspectives, research increasingly focuses on patient-reported outcomes (PROs). This approach ensures that the experiences and priorities of individuals with fibromyalgia are central to research design, assessment, and treatment evaluation.

Multidisciplinary Care Models: The exploration of multidisciplinary care models recognizes the diverse nature of fibromyalgia symptoms. Collaborative efforts among healthcare professionals from various disciplines aim to provide holistic and coordinated care, addressing both physical and psychosocial aspects of the condition.

As research advances, individuals with fibromyalgia can look forward to a future with improved diagnostic tools, more effective treatments, and a deeper understanding of the biological and psychosocial aspects of the condition.

Personal Stories of Triumph

Amidst the challenges of fibromyalgia, personal stories of triumph inspire hope and resilience. Individuals who have successfully navigated their fibromyalgia journey share valuable insights, providing encouragement for others facing similar challenges.

Empowerment through Advocacy: Many individuals with fibromyalgia find empowerment through advocacy. Sharing personal stories, participating in awareness campaigns, and actively contributing to the fibromyalgia community fosters a sense of purpose and solidarity.

Success in Symptom Management: Personal stories often highlight successful strategies for symptom management. Whether through medication adjustments, lifestyle changes, or a combination of approaches, these narratives offer practical insights for others seeking ways to enhance their well-being.

Achieving Milestones: Personal triumphs extend beyond symptom management to encompass various life milestones. Individuals share stories of pursuing education, advancing in their careers, and building fulfilling relationships despite the challenges posed by fibromyalgia.

Fostering Resilience: Resilience is a common theme in personal stories of triumph. Individuals emphasize the importance of cultivating resilience, adapting to changes, and finding inner strength to face the ups and downs of living with fibromyalgia.

Building Supportive Networks: Personal narratives often underscore the significance of building supportive networks. Whether through family, friends, or online communities, individuals with fibromyalgia find strength in connecting with others who understand their experiences.

Pursuing Passion and Hobbies: Personal stories frequently highlight the pursuit of passion and hobbies as a source of joy and fulfilment. Engaging in activities that bring a sense of purpose and happiness contributes to a positive outlook despite the challenges of fibromyalgia.

Overcoming Stigma: Triumph over the stigma associated with fibromyalgia is a powerful theme. Individuals share stories of breaking down stereotypes, advocating for understanding, and challenging misconceptions about the condition.

Personal stories of triumph serve as beacons of hope, illustrating that a fulfilling and meaningful life is possible despite the challenges posed by fibromyalgia. These narratives inspire others to persevere and find their own paths to resilience and triumph.

Building a Positive Outlook

Building a positive outlook is an essential aspect of living with fibromyalgia. Cultivating a mindset focused on hope, resilience, and self-care contributes to overall well-being and enhances the ability to navigate the complexities of the condition.

Embracing Mindfulness: Mindfulness practices, such as meditation and mindful breathing, promote a positive outlook by fostering a focus on the present moment. Mindfulness encourages individuals to accept their experiences without judgment, reducing anxiety about the past or future.

Gratitude Practices: Incorporating gratitude practices into daily life involves acknowledging and appreciating positive aspects, no matter how small. Keeping a gratitude journal, reflecting on positive moments, and expressing thanks contribute to a more positive mindset.

Setting Realistic Expectations: Setting realistic expectations involves acknowledging limitations and pacing activities accordingly. Establishing achievable goals and celebrating small victories helps build a positive outlook by fostering a sense of accomplishment.

Seeking Professional Support: When needed, seeking professional support, such as counselling or therapy, can contribute to a positive outlook.

Mental health professionals can provide tools for coping with challenges, managing stress, and enhancing overall emotional well-being.

Focusing on Self-Care: Prioritizing self-care activities contributes to a positive outlook. Whether through relaxation techniques, hobbies, or activities that bring joy, self-care fosters a sense of balance and enhances overall resilience.

Connecting with Supportive Communities: Engaging with supportive communities, whether online or in-person, creates a sense of belonging. Sharing experiences, receiving encouragement, and offering support to others contribute to a positive and uplifting environment.

Celebrating Achievements: Celebrating achievements, no matter how small, is integral to building a positive outlook. Recognizing personal strengths, resilience, and progress fosters a sense of pride and reinforces a positive mindset.

Fostering a Growth Mindset: Adopting a growth mindset involves viewing challenges as opportunities for growth and learning. Embracing the idea that one's abilities can be developed over time contributes to a positive and forward-looking perspective.

Acknowledging Emotional Responses: Acknowledging and validating emotional responses to fibromyalgia challenges is an important aspect of building a positive outlook.

Allowing oneself to experience and process emotions without judgment contributes to emotional well-being.

Building a positive outlook is a continuous process that involves intentional practices, self-reflection, and the cultivation of a mindset that embraces resilience and hope. By incorporating these strategies, individuals with fibromyalgia can navigate their journey with a sense of optimism and empowerment.

Advances in research, personal stories of triumph, and strategies for building a positive outlook collectively contribute to a comprehensive perspective on living with fibromyalgia. By embracing the potential for progress, drawing inspiration from personal narratives, and cultivating a positive mindset, individuals can navigate their fibromyalgia journey with resilience and hope for a brighter future.

Chapter 15: Your Fibromyalgia Journey

As individuals embark on their fibromyalgia journey, Chapter 15 serves as a practical guide to personal empowerment and ongoing well-being. This chapter focuses on setting personal goals, monitoring progress, and emphasising the importance of continuing self-care practices beyond the information provided in the book.

Setting Personal Goals

Setting personal goals is a foundational step in managing fibromyalgia effectively. Goals provide a sense of direction, motivation, and a framework for individuals to actively participate in their own well-being. Tailoring goals to personal aspirations and the unique challenges of fibromyalgia fosters a proactive and empowering approach.

Identifying Priorities: Begin by identifying priorities and areas of life that hold significance. Whether it's improving physical fitness, managing stress, enhancing sleep quality, or pursuing personal interests, understanding what matters most helps shape meaningful goals.

Setting Realistic and Attainable Goals: Realistic and attainable goals are key to success. Consider factors such as current health status, energy levels, and lifestyle constraints when defining goals. Setting small, achievable objectives creates a sense of accomplishment and builds momentum.

Establishing Short-Term and Long-Term Goals: Distinguish between short-term and long-term goals to create a comprehensive plan. Short-term goals focus on immediate objectives, while long-term goals provide a broader perspective and guide sustained efforts over an extended period.

Incorporating Different Life Domains: Fibromyalgia affects various aspects of life, including physical health, mental well-being, relationships, and personal interests. Consider setting goals that encompass these different life domains, ensuring a holistic approach to self-improvement.

Prioritising Self-Care: Prioritising self-care is a fundamental goal in managing fibromyalgia. This may involve incorporating relaxation techniques, establishing a consistent sleep routine, and engaging in activities that bring joy and relaxation.

Seeking Professional Guidance: When establishing health-related goals, seek input from healthcare providers. Collaborating with medical professionals ensures that goals align with individual health needs and are safe and appropriate for the specific challenges posed by fibromyalgia.

Adjusting Goals as Needed: Fibromyalgia symptoms can fluctuate, necessitating flexibility in goal setting. Be prepared to adjust goals based on changes in health status, energy levels, and other factors. Adaptability ensures continued progress and prevents feelings of discouragement.

Setting personal goals empowers individuals to actively shape their fibromyalgia journey, fostering a sense of control and purpose in the face of challenges.

Monitoring Progress

Monitoring progress is an essential component of goal-oriented fibromyalgia management. Regular assessment allows individuals to track achievements, identify areas for improvement, and make informed adjustments to their self-care strategies.

Tracking Physical Health: For goals related to physical health, monitoring can involve keeping a record of symptoms, energy levels, and any changes in pain intensity. Utilising symptom journals or health tracking apps facilitates accurate and ongoing assessment.

Assessing Mental Well-Being: Mental well-being is integral to overall health.

Assessing mood, stress levels, and emotional responses provides insight into the impact of self-care practices on mental health. Identifying patterns helps refine strategies for managing psychological aspects of fibromyalgia.

Evaluating Sleep Quality: Sleep plays a crucial role in fibromyalgia management. Individuals can monitor sleep patterns, quality of sleep, and any factors that may impact sleep hygiene. This information informs adjustments to bedtime routines and sleep-related goals.

Reviewing Lifestyle Changes: Lifestyle modifications, such as dietary changes or exercise routines, can be monitored by tracking adherence to the plan and noting any associated changes in symptoms or overall well-being.

Regular review guides the refinement of lifestyle strategies.

Reflecting on Achievements: Celebrate achievements, no matter how small. Regularly reflecting on progress reinforces a positive mindset and encourages continued efforts. Acknowledging accomplishments builds motivation and resilience.

Seeking Feedback: Consider seeking feedback from healthcare providers, support networks, or professionals involved in specific aspects of the fibromyalgia journey. External perspectives can provide valuable insights and contribute to a more comprehensive understanding of progress.

Adjusting Strategies: If monitoring reveals challenges or areas for improvement, be willing to adjust strategies. This may involve revisiting goals, refining self-care practices, or seeking additional support as needed. Flexibility is key to ongoing progress.

Recognizing Non-linear Progress: The fibromyalgia journey often involves non-linear progress. Individuals may experience fluctuations in symptoms and well-being. Recognizing that progress may have ups and downs helps maintain a realistic and compassionate perspective.

Monitoring progress is a dynamic and ongoing process that empowers individuals to actively engage with their fibromyalgia management, fostering a sense of agency and adaptability.

Continuing Self-Care Beyond the Book

The journey with fibromyalgia extends beyond the information provided in the book, emphasizing the importance of cultivating a sustainable and lifelong commitment to self-care. Chapter 15 encourages individuals to integrate self-care practices into their daily lives, promoting long-term well-being.

Integrating Self-Care into Routine: Self-care should be integrated seamlessly into daily routines. This may involve setting aside dedicated time for relaxation, exercise, or other self-care activities. Consistency fosters the habituation of self-care practices.

Exploring Holistic Approaches: Consider exploring holistic approaches to self-care that address the physical, mental, and emotional aspects of well-being. Engage in activities that nurture overall health, such as mindfulness practices, holistic therapies, and activities that bring joy.

Building a Supportive Environment: Surrounding oneself with a supportive environment is integral to sustained self-care. Communicate openly with family, friends, and healthcare providers about needs and challenges. Foster relationships that contribute positively to well-being.

Staying Informed: Stay informed about new developments in fibromyalgia management, research, and support resources.

Being aware of emerging information empowers individuals to make informed decisions and adapt their self-care strategies based on the latest insights.

Connecting with the Fibromyalgia Community: The fibromyalgia community offers a valuable source of support and shared experiences. Continue to connect with individuals who understand the challenges of fibromyalgia, whether through local support groups, online forums, or community events.

Revisiting Goals Periodically: Periodically revisit personal goals to ensure they align with current priorities and health status. Adjust goals as needed, and set new objectives that reflect evolving aspirations.

This ongoing process ensures that self-care remains tailored to individual needs.

Prioritizing Flexibility: Recognize the need for flexibility in self-care practices. Fibromyalgia symptoms may vary, and life circumstances can change. Being adaptable and willing to modify self-care strategies ensures continued relevance and effectiveness.

Cultivating a Positive Mindset: Cultivate a positive mindset as a foundational aspect of ongoing self-care. Embrace resilience, celebrate achievements, and approach challenges with a sense of empowerment. A positive outlook contributes significantly to overall well-being.

Balancing Rest and Activity: Striking a balance between rest and activity is crucial for individuals with fibromyalgia. Periods of rest should be integrated into daily routines, and activities should be paced to prevent overexertion. This balance contributes to sustained energy and symptom management.

Continuing self-care beyond the information provided in the book is a lifelong commitment. By integrating personalized, holistic, and adaptable self-care practices, individuals can navigate their fibromyalgia journey with resilience, well-being, and a sense of empowerment.

In conclusion, Chapter 15 serves as a guide for individuals navigating their fibromyalgia journey. Setting personal goals, monitoring progress, and emphasizing ongoing self-care beyond the book provide a comprehensive framework for active participation in well-being. As individuals engage with these principles, they are empowered to shape their fibromyalgia journey with intention, adaptability, and a commitment to long-term health and happiness.

Conclusion: Navigating Your Fibromyalgia Journey with Empowerment and Hope

In concluding "The Complete Fibromyalgia Guide for Women," we acknowledge the profound challenges that individuals with fibromyalgia face daily and the resilience required to navigate this complex journey. This comprehensive guide has sought to provide not only information but a roadmap for empowerment, understanding, and the cultivation of hope.

Throughout these fifteen chapters, we have delved into the intricacies of fibromyalgia, offering insights into its origins, impact on women's health, and the myriad factors that contribute to its complexity. From medical approaches to lifestyle modifications, mental health considerations, and the unique challenges faced by women, each chapter has aimed to equip readers with knowledge to make informed decisions about their health.

We explored the importance of relationships, support networks, and strategies for managing the unique challenges women encounter throughout different stages of life. Addressing the intersection of fibromyalgia with the menstrual cycle, pregnancy, and menopause, we recognized the need for tailored approaches to care.

The guide ventured into the realms of advocacy, research, and the promising future outlook for fibromyalgia. We celebrated personal triumphs and the resilience demonstrated by individuals who have navigated the complexities of fibromyalgia with courage and determination.

In the concluding chapter, we emphasized the significance of setting personal goals, monitoring progress, and the enduring commitment to self-care beyond the book. This final chapter encapsulates the essence of empowerment, encouraging individuals to actively shape their fibromyalgia journey with intention, adaptability, and a dedication to long-term well-being.

As we close this comprehensive guide, it is essential to recognize that the fibromyalgia journey is unique to each individual. There is no one-size-fits-all approach, and the strategies explored in this book are meant to be adaptable, personalised, and continually evolving.

Above all, we extend a message of hope. Hope for advancements in research that may unveil new treatment modalities and approaches. Hope for individuals to find strength and inspiration in personal stories of triumph. Hope for a future where awareness, understanding, and support for fibromyalgia continue to grow.

Remember that the journey with fibromyalgia is not defined by the challenges alone but by the resilience, courage, and strength demonstrated in overcoming them. Each day presents an opportunity for growth, self-discovery, and the pursuit of a fulfilling life despite the obstacles.

As you embark on your fibromyalgia journey, carry with you the knowledge gained from these pages, but more importantly, carry the spirit of empowerment and hope.

You are not alone, and your journey is marked by the potential for progress, triumphs, and a future where fibromyalgia is better understood and effectively managed.

Wishing you strength, resilience, and a future filled with hope on your unique fibromyalgia journey.